Table of Contents

Prelude

Calendars

Journaling/Writing

Healthy Recipes/Snacks

Healthy Activities

Glossary

Additional Resources, References &

Citations

Prelude

I don't by any means attempt to force my way on others when it comes to anything holistic, but! I HIGHLY RECOMMEND the following to help promote balance:

1. If you are going **consume meat** to do so in moderation or not at all.

2. JOURNAL about what you are doing **mentally, physically, spiritually** as often as possible.

That being said, I have included a list of **healthy activities** that can assist in helping to bring you back to balance along with meal and snack **ideas and activities** to help your body get back to a HIGHER VIBRATION. I've also included a step by step guide to get **the writer in you** started in the process of getting your thoughts down on paper, even if it is just a sentence or two so you can get used to writing often. I've had the **idea** for this book for a long time and am finally getting a moment to get the ideas to print-so it doesn't look **aesthetically perfect** but the content is definitely well worth using in your **journey to healing and/or balance**. I am a gifted interpretative dancer and the production of this particular piece definitely reflects the artist in me. You will notice through-out the book bolded/highlighted and colored ETCETERA words, which are definitely meant to catch your attention. I'm sure once I get into the swing of things **my writings** in the future will appear to be much prettier and clean cut, but in the meantime know that being a **holistic-minded person** doesn't mean being **perfect**, it means doing what it takes to get yourself back to balance when your life circumstances throw you a **curve ball**. When those frustrating unpredictable things happen like they always manage to at the most inopportune time causing you MENTAL, PHYSICAL, SPIRITUAL distress, **pull out the handy dandy** and come along with me on the journey to healing and discovery of peace & balance. As you begin to follow the guidance and suggestions offered to you in the handy dandy holistic guide and workbook you'll see the more evolved YOU, and MOST IMPORTANTLY...Have FUN!

I humbly dedicate this book to my little ray of sunshine & hope Naailah Sarai who is a vegetarian and one of my besties from high school's eldest child Amber Jeanette who passed away in 2015 after having committed to becoming vegan, fly high sweetheart!!!

CALENDARS

Calendar-(2015-2017)

(2015)

(2016)

(2017)

ANOTHER THING I HIGHLY recommend as you move along in your journey to wellness is to keep as many **calendars** around as possible. I believe in this so much so that I'm often caught giving them as gifts. When I say calendars I mean **planners, desk and wall calendars**, and even those **little pocket sized calendars for your purse or briefcase**. I used the illustration above to emphasize the need for short and long term calendars to WRITE **details** about goals and plans that are fast approaching and also up to 5 years OR MORE in the future. It's also a good idea to have **different size** boxes with which to write notes in, the small boxes work for little details but the large ones can really pack a punch with keeping you on track with your list of **goals and/or PLANS**.

SO GET THOSE CALENDARS OUT AND GET

TO PLANNING!!!

Journaling vs. notetaking

This way of keeping a journal is for the "**non writer-beginning writing**" I.E. a person who is not into writing much, this will ask you to take note of things so you can look back to reflect

THE "NON-WRITER"

The beauty of **JOURNALING is** that no one has to see it but you so it **doesn't need to** be revised or edited (and if you keep one in a private place and/or a lock on it, it can be like a personal diary that you use to vent in etc...). You'll want to use this section of the handy dandy guidebook to get into the habit of **simply putting your thoughts down daily, even if it is only one sentence or so.** This practice will help you to get into a rhythm and also give you a chance to take a **quick breather from the hustle and bustle of everyday life**. Use your time journaling to **reflect on dietary choices, interactions** with potentially TOXIC people and/or balancing VS DYSFUNCTIONAL- ADDICTIVE **behaviors**. Those reflections can help you to make necessary adjustments to pull you back to a more grounded and balanced state of mind.

SEE EXAMPLES

Mon- MEMORIAL DAY -   OFF WORK JUST RELAXED AND STAYED AROUND THE HOUSE.

Tues-   TODAY I WENT TO AN APPOINTMENT AND IT WENT Rather SMOOTHLY COMPARED TO OTHER TIMES @ THIS PLACE. I HAD MY USUAL CUP OF COFFEE THEN HEADED TO THE LIBRARY Afterwards.

Wed-

Thurs- I DIDN'T HAVE TIME TO WRITE YESTERDAY WITH SCHOOL/WORK/KID... WAAAY TO BUSY THESE DAYS

Fri-

Sat-

Sun-

Your Turn to Write

use this section to write notes/memos/brief reflections everyday if possible··· don't worry if you forget to check in on a particular day, just get this book back out and have at it the next day–if you feel inspired, write more, if not so much then write less– no pressure!!!

Mon-

Tues-

Wed-

Thurs-

Fri-

Sat-

Sun-

Mon-

Tues-

Wed-

Thurs-

Fri-

Sat-

Sun-

Mon-

Tues-

Wed-

Thurs-

Friday-

Saturday-

Sunday-

JOURNALS

This section is for actual writing with more details/description

For the Intermediate-Advanced Writers

As you get used to journaling more frequently, move into this section and begin to add **MORE DETAILS** about your day. Even if you only work on it a **few times per week** you will begin to think of **more details** to **reflect** on which can give you clues about how to proceed with the process of getting yourself back to **BALANCE**. Journaling on this level could lead to the writing of a memoir

or other similar types of writing that you may eventually want to **publish and/or** at least share.

With others. While this type of journaling is similar to the above, **it goes one step further** and includes more **details and reflections** for the days that entries are added.

*SEE EXAMPLES *

Date: Tuesday December 11, 2015

Entry #1 I woke up after a night of tossing and turning, worrying about what I was going to do about my issues with my room-mate. She made it clear that she is interested in something other than friendship but I am not and would never be. I have been frantically searching for a new place, attempting to find the best possible place for myself and my 4 year old. Between school and work and working on my writing, I've been preoccupied enough... also, exhausted from thinking too much after school, subbing all over the city and my 4 year olds daycare issues that pop up at the worst possible times... my brain needs to rest.

Date: Wednesday December 12, 2015

Entry #2: I spent the entire first six or so months that I was staying with this lune cleaning up the wretched mess from sink loads of dishes, cat vomit and fur everywhere and also cooking and cleaning, in addition to paying rent! I guess if I was a left brained introvert (both of which I can relate to and is actually why we were friends to begin with) with few friends and in depression who doesn't even have custody of her own kid because she lacks a nurturing side I'd want an experienced holistic educator to stay on as my mate and continue to fix my life up too. I would have been willing to stay as a friend, but IM NOT GAY!! And she started making romantic advances at me and that is where I draw the line. So here I am in yet another pickle attempting to get myself and my kid to safety while I search for a better living situation than the very wild neighborhood I moved from when my lease was up last year. That is the type of place that I qualify for right now and I've been hesitant to move back to something like that anytime soon, BUT I WILL ... it would be a lot easier if she weren't forcing me out LITERALLY A FEW weeks before I'm expecting a good lump sum of money to at least pay for a hotel and/or RV with (which is my plan temporarily until I can get a decent place) What an awful person she has to be inside to think this is ok to do to a single mother unnecessarily. I will not let karma deal with her and continue to hold onto hope and keep it moving though because I don't want nor have time to fight w/ imbalanced sociopaths. I thought I'd make this section a bit spicy to keep you reading... nothing like reading someone else's dirt.

Date: Thursday December 13, 2015

Entry #3: I woke up twice this morning, once on my own because my body clock is used to waking at that time, then to my dysfunctional roommate decided to text me about some crap leaking in the fridge. Instead of just asking me to clean the fridge, she puts a hole in a baggie and has me clean it up. When I arrived here she was controlling and didn't take very good care of this house at all. She was/is an opportunist and will reap what she sows for attempting to take advantage of my situation. She suddenly broke up with her boyfriend and then commenced to control my every move. She wanted far more than to help someone in need of a friend and to give them a chance while they get their life together. I paid this woman with sweat equity when I got here yet she took it upon herself to ask for more. I always assume the best and give people the benefit of the doubt, but she is a very sick and disgusting person who needs to be humbled. She doesn't have her kid because the thought of taking care of another human life is miserable to her, yet she has two cats that she lets climb all over her kitchen table and vomit all over the place. What a miserable life she must have to love and desire the company of her animals over her own child's. Not only must she be miserable but she has to be the most self-centered ego-centric person to be so selfish towards her own, I've heard her on several occasions refuse affection to her child and also act like a complete cold-hearted psyho-path to her. As I write I'm realizing that t I have nothing a thing to envy in her (as I had already concluded) but she has much. She lives a cold, miserable life, thanks to her similar mother who based on her description was not much different than she as a mother. She thinks money and status buys love and happiness, perhaps that is the lesson that I can take from this situation.

Date: Friday December 14, 2015

Entry #4: I'm starting to realize that everyone thinks I must be crazy for having left my well off ex-husband and then a few years later to go and join a church that some have referred to as a cult. When you are raised in so much insanity with drinking, drugs and sexual dysfunction and you are quite aware that something is not quite right and there must be something better out there, then you find a place that teaches you to avoid all of the above and to love and cherish your family....you tend to lean towards that group of folks/way of living. I was very active in that church for nearly a decade until my now grown kids turned into teenagers in high school and started walking away from it themselves. I stayed connected with them for a while but when I moved back to my old neighborhood and was not able to tolerate being around a few self-righteous holier than thou sort of folks who participated in gossip and made presumptions about things they knew nothing about, I was pretty much ousted. I am so glad that I got myself pulled together after that period of my life. I have been trying to get some things in place for nearly a decade now that could help all of humanity... I'm starting to wonder if it is a futile effort.... Like some of my relatives, there are SOME who seem to want to stay asleep, dysfunctional, sick and uninterested in helping to heal not only themselves, but the world. I'm not the crazy one and but I'm glad that I'm aware of it, but I need to remember to connect with like-minded folks more often because the sickness of those I'm around feels me like sheer insanity. There are definitely some friends in the church, but far too many helps me see why the God of Abraham kept flooding and destroying the inhabitants of earth when he started his communication with humanity. Be sure to keep entries like this in a locked journal unless you want to risk someone trying to sneak and read it, especially if it has lots of information that you' prefer not share ☺

Your Turn To Write Again.....

Use this section to write more extensive notes to

yourself and/or others about events etc....

This time give more detailed reflections everyday

if possible and don't worry if you forget to check

in on a particular day, just get this book-or your

own journal if you have decided to invest in one

at this point, and have at it the next day!!

Date:

Entry #:

Date:

Entry #:

Date:

Entry #:

Date:

Entry #:

Date:

Entry #:

Date:

Entry #:

Date:

Entry #:

Date:

Entry #:

Date:

Entry #:

Date:

Entry #

My Fav Holistic Recipes

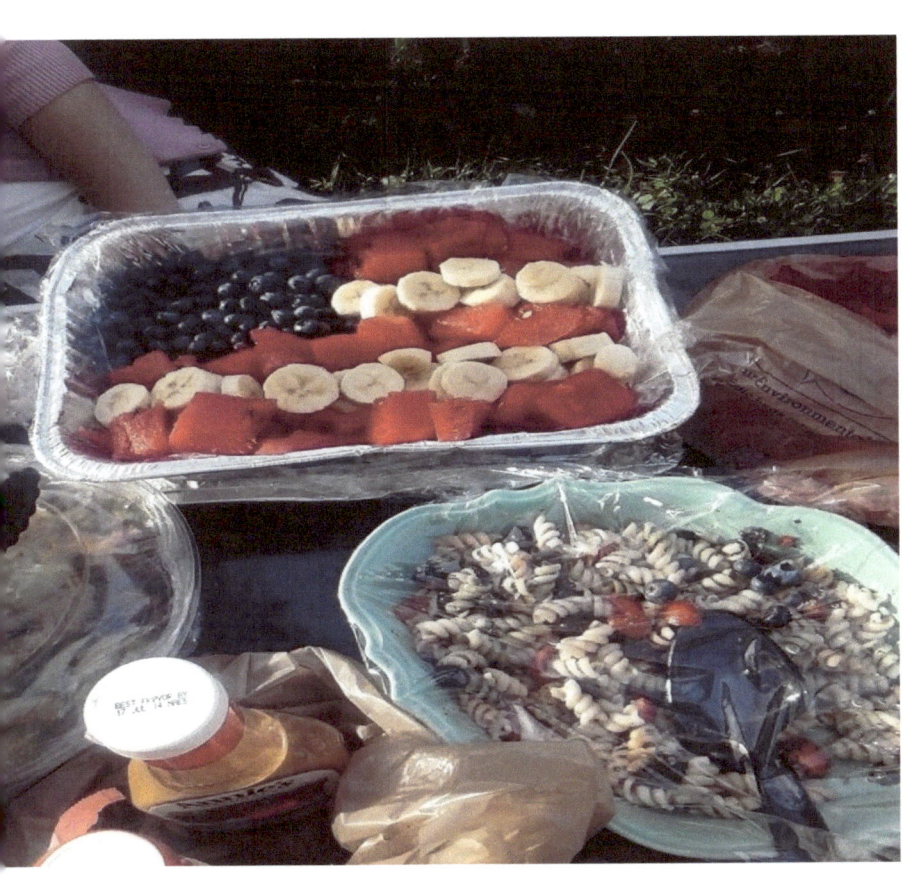

I decided to include **some of my favorite recipes** and/or dishes to give my readers a **starting point** for ideas of **healthier/healing food** choices. Since I am only including **SOME** of the recipes, I added some **links to resources at the end of this book** that you can look to for the **recipes for dishes** I mention but don't list. I nannied for a very sweet family from India and learned to prepare many healthy **vegetarian and non-vegetarian recipes**. Additionally, since I am a **pescatarian** and I have a four year old who is a complete **vegetarian**, I decided to share some of our favorite veg **"go to" meals** for anyone trying to **ease up on meat consumption**. While I was working on this book I was **taking**

classes, working as a sub-teacher, and taking care of my 4-year old, so I sometimes was **forced to eat in a hurry.** I've included veggie swaps I made when that would happen because I definitely **DON'T recommend eating too much fast food** meats. This section gives you a GOOD amount of ideas to build on & even some room to **conjure up some of your own.** If you're in to spicy food, the jalapeno cheeseburgers are a top pick.

I. Curry Chick Peas (Chole)

1-2 cans chick peas
(See LINK for recipe for Masala)

1. Buy or prepare masala

2. Add the chick peas & allow to simmer or cook in a slow cooker.

3. Cook till the beans are tender.

4. Serve over rice or as a chat dish.

II.   Curry Chicken

1-2 lbs. of chicken (cubed thigh or breast pieces) + See link for meat Masala recipe

1. Prepare Masala

2. Add the meat & allow simmering or cooking in a slow cooker till the beans are tender.

3. Serve over rice or as a chat dish

III. **Hummus**

*see kosher/Jewish food isle for instantly ready hummus- just add olive oil-OR GET A CONTAINER OF PREMADE HUMMUS FROM A SPECIALTY SHOP –BC SOMETIMES YA GOTTA TREAT YOURSELF and NOT COOK !

IV. **Pita Pizza**

1-2 bags of whole wheat pita pockets

Homemade or store bought pizza sauce

Mozzarella cheese

Slice pitas in half and top as desired

V. <mark>Veggie Burgers</mark>

1 package Quorn brand veggie burgers

1-2 tomatoes

Smoked provolone or Gouda cheese slices

Head of lettuce

Goddess dressing

Whole wheat buns

Prepare burger as you would a normal hamburger, but you don't need to cook it as long. Be sure to try out different dressings to keep it interesting and moist. Before I went veg, I tried my first veggie burger and could not understand why ANYONE would ever be a vegetarian if this was any indicator of what eating would be like. It was just awful. It tasted like three pieces of bread and had very little intrigue to it. Later, after beginning my vegetarian conversion, I met a few vegan friends who introduced me to the idea of actually adding delicious sauces and even hummus to the burger and maybe even throwing it on a wrap to make it more worth my while. It was at that point that I became convinced that veggie burgers were not the enemy!!! Top that burger with some goodness and dig in!!!

VI. Superliscious sweet potatoes & carrot wraps

½-3/4 lbs. carrots

1-2 large sweet potatoes

Garlic/ginger paste

Smoked provolone cheese

Fresh spinach

Tomatoes, spinach or whole wheat tortilla wraps

Sauté the veggies (except the spinach) in a pan w/ onions/garlic/ginger etc…. then place on top of the tortilla. Be sure to prep the tortilla for all of those yummy veggies with some fresh spinach and your favorite cheese before putting the hot veggies on top and wrapping it up! I've also included chicken breast in this dish in the past for my older kids who were meat eaters.

VII. **Chat**

(See recipe for chole)

Frozen samosa or 1 pkg of prepared papdis

1 of onion

1 bunch cilantro

Indian chutneys (to taste) –tamarind/mint etc...

Place Papdi's or wacked samosa on a large place and layer chole', veggies and chutneys

for a festival in your mouth.

VIII. Gnocchi w/ spinach & mushroom Alfredo sauce

1 bag of frozen gnocchi

1 jar of ready-made or homemade Alfredo sauce

1 bag of fresh or frozen spinach

½ lb. container of mushrooms

Combine all ingredients, simmer and serve over your favorite pasta.

Additional favorite dishes

Brown Stew Fish

Taco Soup

Spinach & Black Bean Quesadillas

Veggie chili cheese fries

Veggie Nachos

Fruit Salad

Pasta Salad

Veggie Fast Food Swaps

Eat on the go a lot? Try some of these swaps, & also see healthy fast food swap ideas in reference section.

MCDONALD'S –Grilled onion cheddar burger (**remove burger**)- SEE IF THEY WILL GO HEAVY ON THE GRILLED ONIONS... IT'S AMAZING

WHITE CASTLE- jalapeno burger w/ **cheese and onions only**

RALLIES- mushroom Swiss burger **without the burger** (they put some sauce on this that makes this a yummy inexpensive veggie option that you can eat on the fly.

TACO BELL- Sub bean for beef on most any MEAT dish

Healthier Comfort Food -Snack Options

WHOLE WHEAT crackers, Olives and cheese, **Veggie** crumbles nachos, Homemade SPINACH dips w/ tons of **spinach**, String cheese, and Fresh fruit, Toast w/ **garden veggie** or **Tofutti** cheese spread, Peanut butter and jelly,BEANburritos, REAL FRUIT Popsicles,**Smoothie**s,Dried fruit, Bowl of cereal, Peanut butter Toast,Pretzels,**Chips & salsa, HUMMUS ON EZEKIAL BREAD**

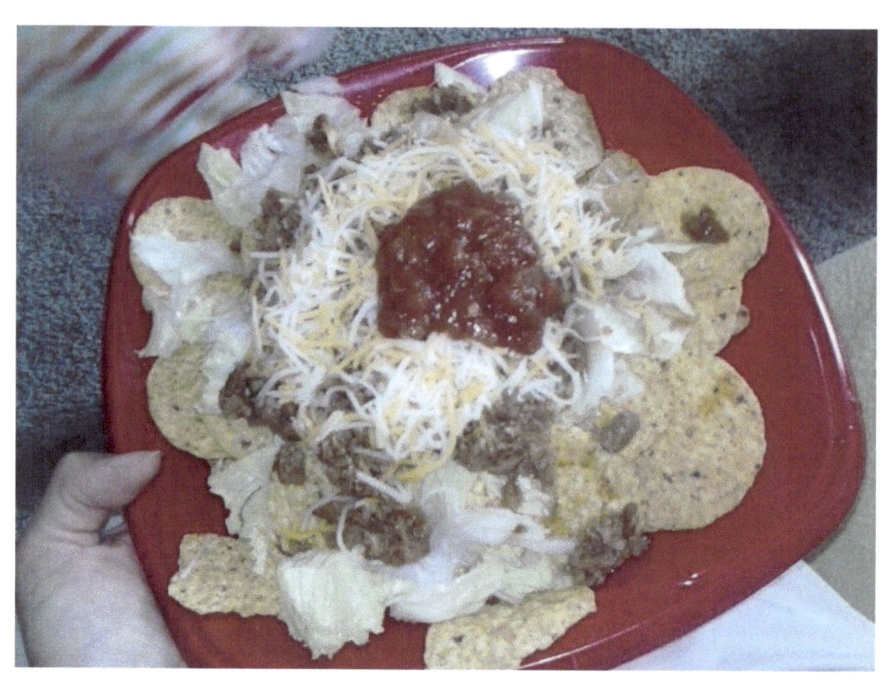

You are what you eat!!

EAT HEALTHIER

NOW

Fill in your own Favorite. Healthy option recipes/snack ideas

I _____

_____

_____

II. _____

III.

IV.

V

.

101 Balancing Activities to Do!

Engage in these activities to balance yourself
instead of dysfunctional behaviors

1. Call a friend 2. WATCH

2. a Netflix movie 3. **Play** a board game with your kid and/or be silly with your pet 4. Eat **some fun/healthy snacks** 5. Eat a piece of **chocolate** or hard candy 6. Watch a **COOKING show** 7. Organize the trunk of your car 8. Put up some fun post on Facebook or send an **ENCOURAGING** email to a loved one 9. **CLEAN** the

bathroom(s) and/or kitchen 10.**Pull weeds** or **PLANT flowers** in your garden 11.Take a **walk** around the block 12.Take a long bike ride 24.**ClEAN** out your car at a car wash 25.Learn how to sew 13.Do a Sudoku puzzles 14. Play online gaming 15.READ some books to your kid(s) 16.Do some **CRAFT projects** with neighborhood kids 17.Take a **RELAXING** shower 18.MAKE some rice crispy treats 19.Go shopping at a dollar store 20.Go for a JOY ride around the city or near a mall 21.LISTEN to your favorite MUSIC 22.Ask someone to go for a WALK with you 23.READ OR LISTEN to a favorite book on CD 26.Go petal boating or canoeing 27.Organize your computer documents/files 28.Wax your excess bodily hairs and/or give yourself a manicure and pedicure 29.Try out a new hairstyle 30.**Walk** around the mall 31.**Chew mints** and/or gum 32.Do a **jigsaw puzzle** 33.Follow your breath! 34.Drink a milkshake or smoothie 35.Look through cookbooks for ideas 36.Do the dishes and/or dusting 37.Take a cat nap 38.**Exercise** 39.**Hug** someone you love40.Clean out the oven and/or fridge41.**Write out/plan something constructive** to do w/your time like a new hobby or volunteer work42.**Spend some of the money** you saved by NOT doing the dysfunctional things43.Eat some ALL NATURAL FRUIT icecream44.**BALANCE** your checkbook45.Check a book out at the **LIBRARY** 46.Read a comic book or magazine47.**Play with a stress** ball48.Plan a staycation or vacation49.Spend time grooming yourself50.**CALL A LOVED ONE** 51.Brush and floss your teeth52.SPEND TIME with your close FRIENDS OR FAMILY 53.**GIVE YOURSELF** a **treat** every day you have successfully done something other than A DYSFUNCTIONAL behavior

54.**Dance** in the store 55.Go to a local special event 56.Play solitaire or something else 57.**CREATE** a family tree 58.Have a quick chat with the mail person 59.Make a **dinner reservation** at a favorite restaurant 60.**PLAY** an instrument 61 Visit/**VOLUNTEER** at a daycare 62.Revisit your motivations for why you don't want to smoke/drink/overeat.. 63.Take silly pictures64.**Create** a scrapbook65.Do some IMPROVEMENTS on your house66.Write in a **JOURNAL** 67.Clean out yourbasement/closets68.Org anize your containers of pictures69.Gohiking70.**Org anize** your CD's in whatever order fits you best71.Take a bubble BATH72.**Watch birds73**.Take a quick road trip74.Do a load of laundry75.**Eat** a **healthy snack76.**Go swimming **77.PLANT** some spices78.Fix up your car79.**Search the internet for something new to LEARN/STUDY 80.RUN** on a treadmill**81.CLEAN** up your neighborhood 82.**Write** some poetry83.Go SKATING84Go shopping in a small town85.Eat some frozen **custard86Go to a batting cage87Go** sledding88.Scrub yourcar89.Drink some herbal tea90.**Kiss** your mate91.Go skydiving92.**GET HEALING ENERGY** work and/or a **MASSAGE** 93.Organize your desk94.**ORGANIZE** your storage space(s)95.Go to an dollar movie96.**Trim the weeds**97.**RIDE A BIKE** in the woods or park98.Go to an ice-cream shop99.**TAKE PICTURES** of the sunset 100. Make greeting cards and treat bags for various people to say thanks and/or I'm thinking of you

101 Start a MINI NOTEBOOK that contains a list of things you are grateful for!!

Your Favorite Balancing Activities

*Describe here what you can do "or did" in place of
dysfunctional/unhealthy activities .....*

1._____

_____

_____

_____

_____

2._____

_____

_____

_____

_____

3._____

_____

_____

_____

_____

_____

_____

4._____

_____

_____

_____

5._____

_____

_____

_____

_____

_____

_____

_____

_____

_____

Glossary

1. **CHAAT** – (Hindi/Nepali: चाट, Urdu/Punjabi: چاٹ) is a term describing savory snacks, typically served at road-side tracks from stalls or food carts in India, Pakistan, Nepal and Bangladesh.[1] [2] With its origins in Uttar Pradesh, [3] chaat has become immensely popular in the rest of South Asia. The word derives from Hindi cāṭ चाट (tasting, a delicacy),

from *caṭnā* चाटना (*to lick*),
from <u>Prakritcaṭṭei</u> चट्टेइ (*to devour
with relish, eat noisily*).[4 2.
CHOLE'– *bhature* (Hindi: छोले भट्टूरे,
Punjabi: ਛੋਲੇ ਭਟੂਰੇ), *is a combination of
chana masala (spicy chick peas) and
fried bread called bhatoora (made of
maida ALSO: Chana masala* ['tʃəna:
mə'sa:la:], *also known
as* **chole** *masala or channay or
Chholay (plural) is a popular dish in
Indian and
Pakistancuisine.***3.HOLISTIC***– The
holistic concept in* <u>medical
practice</u>, *which is distinct from
the concept in the alternative*

medicine, upholds that all aspects of people's needs including psychological, physical and social should be taken into account and seen as a whole**4.INTRODUCT** Introversion is "the state of or tendency toward being wholly or predominantly concerned with and interested in one's own mental life".[4] Introverts are typically more reserved or reflective.[5] Some popular psychologists have characterized introverts as people whose energy tends to expand through reflection and dwindle during interaction.[6] This is similar to Jung's view, although he focused on mental energy rather than physical energy. Few modern conceptions make this distinction.**5MASALA**Any of various mixtures of spices that are used in South Asian cuisine.

6.PESCATARIANA person whose diet is primarily vegetarian but also includes fish. Also called pesco-vegetarian.**7.LEFT- brained** – Broad generalizations are often made in "pop" psychology about one side or the other having characteristic labels, such as "logical" for the left side or "creative" for the right. These labels are not supported by studies on lateralization, as lateralization does not add specialized usage from either hemisphere.[4] Both hemispheres contribute to both kinds of processes,[5] and experimental evidence provides little support for correlating the structural differences between the sides with such broadly defined functional differences.[6]**8.TOFUTTI-**

Aside from the icecream substitute, the Tofutti brand also produces soybased sour cream, creamcheese, sliced cheese, and "Better than Ricotta" ricotta cheese, in additio n to several entrees suchas a dair yfree pizza. 'Cuties' or 'Tofutti Cut ies', their version of the ice cream sandwich, has avariety of flavors such as vanilla, chocolate, mint chocolate chip and others.

9. VEGETARIAN – One who consumes a diet mostly
consisting of vegetables and fruit only , but usually including
milk, cheese, eggs, etcetera...

(http://www.thefreedictionary.com/https://en.wikipedia.org/wiki/Main_Page)

Additional Resources, References & Citations

1. Things to Do Besides Smoking. (n.d.). Retrieved December 29, 2015, from http://www.determinedtoquit.com/stayingtobaccofree/thingstodobesidessmoking

http://www.determinedtoquit.com/stayingtobaccofree/thingstodobesidessmoking

2. Dictionary, Encyclopedia and Thesaurus. (n.d.). Retrieved December 29, 2015, from http://www.thefreedictionary.com/

   TheFreeDictionary.com:

3. (n.d.). Retrieved December 29, 2015, from https://en.wikipedia.org/wiki/Main_Page

   https://en.wikipedia.org/wiki/Main_Page

4. Eat This, Not That! No-Diet Weight Loss, Nutrition Tips and More | Eat This Not That. (2015, March 24). Retrieved December 29, 2015, from http://www.eatthis.com

   www.eatthis.com

www.ingramcontent.com/pod-product-compliance
Lightning Source LLC
Chambersburg PA
CBHW050814290526
45792CB00001B/118